DOMICILIARY
CHIROPODY

A beginner's guide

DOMICILIARY CHIROPODY

A beginner's guide

by

Alan Whitby

Illustrated by the author

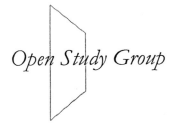

Open Study Group

Copyright © A R Whitby 2002

First edition published 1994 by
OSG Publications
56 Pardown
Oakley
Hampshire
RG23 7DZ

Revised edition published 2002 by
Open Study Group Ltd
Llys Myrddin
Efailwen
Clynderwen
Carmarthenshire
SA66 7XG

ISBN: 1-904406-07-6

Printed in Great Britain by Open Study Group Ltd

Preface to the Revised Edition

Since this book was first published in 1994, there have been some changes affecting self-employed chiropodists. The sections on domiciliary cases, drills and telephones have therefore been updated. The chapter on accounting now includes the Inland Revenue's self assessment procedures, and the section on sterilisation and disinfection has been extensively rewritten. Apart from the odd word here and there all other sections remain unchanged.

CONTENTS

Introduction 9

Advantages and Disadvantages 11

The Right Equipment 15
    The domiciliary case 16
    The drill 18
    Instruments and their sterilisation 20
    Sterilisation and disinfection 22
    Padding and strapping 28
    Materia medica 30
    Looking the part 32

Handling Patients 35
    The telephone 35
    The visit 39
    Patient care and conversation 43
    Broken appointments 46
    Personal safety 47

Practice Management 49
    Obtaining patients 49
    Keeping patients 56
    Accounts 60

Introduction

Nearly all chiropodists who have trained for the private sector will start with a domiciliary practice. Some will never do anything else. Even those who establish flourishing surgeries may still need to consider some home visiting, simply to meet the needs of the local community.

Many NHS facilities for the aged and housebound are undermanned and underfunded. The public still regularly turns to private chiropodists who *will* come to the home, and who *will* spend the required amount of time to treat them properly.

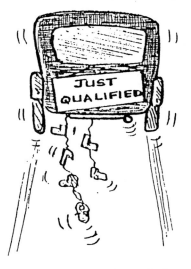

When the writer started down this particular road, he personally felt that he would have benefited greatly from some independent advice on equipment and general practice management; something that would cut its way through the maze of advice supplied by parties with vested interests – often to sell you things!

So the aim of this work is to present an independent overview of what is involved to succeed as a domiciliary chiropodist, both financially and in terms of work satisfaction. It will cover how to secure and keep patients, the basic equipment, a review of basic procedures for professional practice, and also how to handle the business side of things. As such it must be stressed at the outset that much of what follows is deliberately pitched at those who have recently qualified. The longer we have been in practice the more we evolve our own style and preferences. We know what works for us, what we prefer, and the more set in our ways we become. However, it is good for even the seasoned practitioner to consider how others handle things. Positively, there may just be something there that we had not considered. Negatively, it may convince us even more strongly that we've got it right! And if we got it right, and he got it wrong, then why not put our experience in print as well for the benefit of the profession?

Here then is one person's beginner's guide to successful domiciliary chiropody.

Advantages and Disadvantages

There is a fairly old adage:

> Some have cold feet
> some acquire cold feet
> and others have cold feet thrust upon them.

As to why anyone should choose to become a chiropodist is outside the remit of this work. But very soon after making that choice, one has to consider what type of practice it is going to be.

Will it be a fully-equipped podiatrist's surgery? Will it be a domiciliary practice? Will it be a combination of the two? In some cases 'market forces' may dictate. If there are already well-established surgeries covering the community, but a great lack of visiting services, then common sense dictates that, like it or not, that is where the need is. Where the need is, is where the work is!

Surgery work and domiciliary work have their own plusses and minuses. First then, what are the advantages of a domiciliary practice.

1.   You can limit the extent of your practice if you wish. You are not tied to pre-advertised hours in one place. As long as you obtain the volume of patients you need you can then pick and choose your working hours to suit your situation.

     This is why most chiropodists currently working part-time choose visiting work. The term 'part-timer' has been used pejoratively on many occasions, but it must be acknowledged that many now in full-time practice originally worked part-time as their practice built up. There are many who have other responsibilities at present – a young family for example – who only want to work part-time at this stage of their lives. As long as the practitioner is qualified, insured to practise, professional in outlook, charges a professional fee and keeps the Inland Revenue happy, then who should criticise? Certainly domiciliary work suits this kind of practice far more readily than a surgery.

1.   To a great extent you can limit the scope of your practice. You have far more freedom to easily pick and choose your patients and

the level of your practice. Every training scheme has its limitations. The most qualified podiatrist is not going to be a very good brain surgeon! So accept the limitations and boundaries of your own training. If you are not qualified to handle certain situations, or most important, your association's insurance does not cover you for such situations, then you have the perfectly legitimate way out: refer people to a surgery, where there can be better equipment, better aseptic procedures, and – yes – practitioners who may have a greater field of practice and expertise. There is nothing wrong at all in becoming very good in a limited field, but referring elsewhere anything outside that field. People respect that, and *will still come back to you* for their basic treatment. But *you* decide from your own training and feelings what level that is going to be! If you are just starting out in practice and feel overly nervous about any given situation, then again until you get the confidence, or go on that special course, you can refer people to a surgery. With domiciliary work *you* choose!

2. Overheads are much cheaper. To equip a surgery properly is a very large capital investment. It attracts problems like planning permission, business rates, and in some areas, special licences. There will be a very large capital outlay before any patient has walked through the door. If the locals are initially slow about making the journey much will still have to be paid as an ongoing situation. For domiciliary work, once you have your basic equipment, the main outlay will be the running costs of a vehicle.

3. For some the visiting practice suits their temperament. Some people like the 'freedom' to be out and about. Being stuck in a surgery is the kind of working environment they wanted to get away from, especially if they have made a career change to chiropody.

The matter of temperament and personal preference is all important, because some of the above advantages could just as easily be viewed as disadvantages by others. But there are certain problems associated with domiciliary work that you must take on board.

1. You must accept that you really are limited in what you can do in someone's front room – particularly in some of the front rooms

you will encounter! If you have ambitions to be the local King of cryosurgery, Queen of biomechanics, or guru of sporthotics, then very soon you will want a fully-equipped surgery! Even some very basic complaints like verrucae may be uneconomic for both patient and practitioner if a course of chemical cautery is contemplated.

2. It is physically far more tiring to travel to patients rather than have them travel to you. It is also far more taxing to deal with chairs of varying heights, and at the homes of elderly people lugging the furniture around (and sometimes the patient with it) before you start. We will deal briefly with operator's stools under THE VISIT, but if you suffer from any kind of back trouble, be warned! If you do not as yet suffer from any kind of back trouble – still be warned! You do not want your professional fees swallowed up by too many visits to your local friendly osteopath or chiropractor.

3. You must be able to drive and your vehicle must be reliable. If the RAC is always towing you home from scenic parts of Britain, then a visiting practice could be a nightmare. Your vehicle should project an aura of reasonable well-being, not be one that you have to park around the corner in embarrassment. The chiropodist who takes his bicycle clips off at the door does not always inspire the greatest confidence...

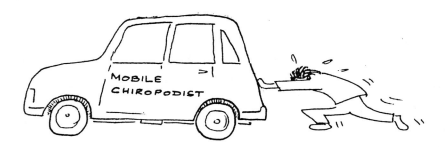

The Right Equipment

The secret of success with domiciliary chiropody is to keep things simple! Often when people start up in practice they go overboard. They panic. What if this or that comes up? – all those nasty rare conditions I've learned about? – I must have all the equipment – just in case... At this vulnerable stage there is always someone around who wants to sell them 'it', and convince them they will come horribly unstuck without 'it'!

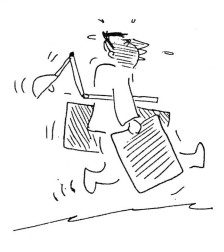

The poor chiropodist then risks a hernia each working day, with great huge cases; and very often finds himself spreading all manner of clutter over the patient's unhygienic carpet, just trying to find the basics he actually needs.

Accept that about 95% of home visiting chiropody is what is commonly called N.C.C. work: that is – Nails, Corns, Callouses. Now consider how little you actually need to care effectively for nails, corns and callouses.

You need certain basic instruments, dressings and medicaments But for 19 out of 20 patients that is *all* you will need! So by all means consider the other 5% and what you might just need. By all means consider what fields you might specialize in – chairside appliance-making for example – but for 95% of patients you will just need the basics. It certainly makes good sense to have extra items in your car, just in case. But as far as the equipment you haul in and out of the car, and in and out of the homes, and up and down stairs – *keep it simple!* You will live a lot longer.

Each practitioner if asked would likely draw up a slightly different list of what he considers the basic essentials. In some respects we all learn by trial and error, and the sensible beginner soon learns what he uses regularly, and what could fittingly be relegated to the car. The prudent beginner also learns that, once he has bought the bare essentials and seen how expensive they are, it is well worth scouring the small ads in the various chiropody journals. As chiropodists retire or some upgrade their equipment, there are often opportunities to buy quality equipment very reasonably second-hand.

In this section then we will consider some basic points on: the case, the drill, our instruments and disinfection/sterilisation of same, padding and strapping, materia medica, and what we wear – looking the part!

The domiciliary case

There are chiropodists who have designed and built their own visiting cases, but the end results often appear heavy and unsatisfactory. If you purchase a case from the usual suppliers there are four main types commercially produced, with variations in between.

1. The original rectangular or square box. This normally opens both at the top and at the side, revealing an instrument panel in a linen holdall, one or two drawers for felts, a holder for dropper bottles, and in older cases a rail to hold loose rolls of strapping. The design flourished for many years. These cases can sometimes be obtained second-hand (making it appear that the fledgling chiropodist has been in practice for thirty years) and variations are still manufactured. However, if you want to use items in modern packaging (e.g. aerosols for disinfection) they do not always fit easily into these older cases.

2. The executive case. Some of these resemble a mitred tool case. They have removable trays, pre-cut foam inserts to hold bottles securely, and at least one popular model has an upright instrument panel with elasticated strips to hold instruments in place. This looks very impressive, although using instruments straight from such a panel raises serious questions about their disinfection. Some allow for all manner of things to be held in foam panels in the lid; one has to then be careful that too many heavier items are not stored in this way, otherwise the whole case can be top-heavy and

overbalance when you open it. Some of these cases are so large that they tempt you to carry far too much with you.

3. The chest of drawers. A more recent style of case opens at the side (in some cases both sides) to reveal a whole series of plastic drawers. This can be ideal if you wish to carry all manner of pre-cut pads. However, if you prefer to carry large sheets of felt and foam and cut each pad individually then you may well need larger and shallower drawers. A plastic chest of drawers may also have the habit of rattling, cracking, or at least looking scratched and sad as the years roll by.

4. The canvass hold-all. A fairly recent addition in the chiropody case market is the canvass haversack, replete with multitudes of compartments, Velcro straps, and a rather hefty price tag. At least one on the market has a small red canvas case attached for the storage of used instruments, which is rather a nice touch. Whether this type of case will help your image as a chiropodist, or give you the appearance of someone about to go hiking in Snowdonia, is a matter of personal taste. Seeing this option, some practitioners have opted for adapting a large vanity case from a department store, for a fraction of the cost. Gentlemen choosing this last option tend to favour the colour black rather than pink.

All the above in their variations have their points, and what you choose is a very personal thing. Someone training for chiropody would do well to carefully examine and handle colleagues' cases, or visit a trade exhibition where the different styles on offer can be inspected. It is a very important purchase and quite an expensive one, and just looking at pictures in a catalogue is not enough to make the right decision for you.

Some cases have a space to hold a domiciliary drill — usually an expensive one distributed by the same supplier. These cases can be very heavy and limit what other things can be carried in them. Two smaller, lighter cases are a lot easier and safer to carry than one big case. Just remember how many times you will be getting in and out of the car and people's homes in a single working day.

The drill

One of the most satisfying conditions to treat in the new patient is onychogryphosis (ram's horn nail). A patient presenting this condition has invariably gone for months, even years, without treatment. The resulting deformity can have serious consequences for their mobility and general equilibrium. The careful use of the drill with a burr or sanding disc to transform years of neglect into something resembling a normal nail, without any discomfort to the patient, is very rewarding.

There are many other situations where the chiropody drill, if not essential, is certainly a very useful part of basic equipment.

As a visiting chiropodist you will obviously want the latest state of the art in portability. You will want effective dust extraction or water jet technology, and a model that runs off a rechargeable unit allowing the full range of power. You will want a lot! It will cost you many hundreds of pounds!

In the real world, most of us have to settle for less initially. All the chiropody suppliers advertise small domiciliary drills, although you can often obtain the same kind of equipment much cheaper by visiting a hobby shop and buying something like a glass engraving kit. As long as you are using the correct chiropody burrs and discs, the drill's origin is immaterial.

The big disadvantage with the cheaper drills is that they do not have provision for dust extraction, and while it is possible to produce your own version from the innards of an old vacuum cleaner this is not really a practical option. So you may well choose to wear a mask each time you use the drill. This Doctor Kildare impersonation looks professional, and shows that you are aware of the dust generated in a normal treatment. Human nail dust infected with trichophyton rubrum has been shown to cause allergies in some people, akin to the symptoms of hay fever. If you fall into that category, wearing a mask may look good, but may not actually give you much real protection. If you wear glasses, with a mask on they will automatically steam up! If you leave the mask off and blow the dust away from you as you work (what a terrible suggestion. . .) – who are you blowing it towards? If nail dust affects you, the only real answer is to purchase expensive equipment with an effective dust extraction or dust dampening system as soon as you can afford it. Even then some nail dust (along with a whole lot more household dust) has to be viewed as an occupational hazard in domiciliary work.

If you are going to use mains power, with the small nail drills make sure that you purchase the appropriate transformer, to allow for sufficient torque and variable speed. You will also need to either carry an extension lead, or permanently extend the lead attached to the transformer. Otherwise the power point will never be near enough. If you work in a depressed area with a large elderly population in homes that have not been rewired since the late 1940's, be prepared to still encounter round pin 15 amp sockets. If there is any danger of this happening, it is worth keeping a square to round pin adaptor in the car. On the rare occasion it is needed, note this down on the patient's card for future reference.

Many chiropodists do away with trailing wires by using battery operated drills.

These allow for greater flexibility of movement, but unless you go up-market with specially rechargeable models you will sacrifice flexibility of speed. The models at the cheaper end of the market will work off standard torch batteries. They normally produce just two speeds. Rechargeable batteries will cut down on expense but you need them fully cooked at the start of each working day, otherwise your two speeds will quickly become 'Slow' and 'Stop'.

Some cheap drills seems to develop dicky switches that inadvertently switch on as the drill rattles around in your case in the car. Opening your case for the worst example of onychogryphosis you have ever seen, you don't want to be greeted by the death rattle of your drill. If there is any possibility of this happening, remove the battery compartment in transit and only reassemble for actual use. And always – repeat always – carry spares!

Instruments and their sterilisation

It is assumed that the reader will not need too much advice on instruments. It is good to check out the different sizes of clippers from a trade rep or at a trade fair to find out what suits your hand size. For heavier work use cantilever nippers to avoid possible strain injuries like tenosynovitis. Do not economise on ingrown nippers; get the very best you can. This writer personally recommends the Thwaites nippers which work on the anvil principle. There is just one cutting edge that meets a flat plane at right angles. This flat plane can be slipped under the offending edge of nail with far less discomfort than with ordinary nippers. Get Blacks files with both rough and fine edges. For dressing scissors, again try out the various sizes. If you are left -handed then get a left-handed pair. They do exist.

As will be stressed later, to avoid any danger of cross infection you actually need a number of sets of these instruments, because their usage is potentially invasive. Even with the best technique in the world, on rare occasions clippers and Blacks files can occasionally cut someone or come in contact with existing breaks in the skin.

If using an autoclave all your instruments will need to be of stainless steel. If they are not they will soon discolour or worse. Be warned too that if you mix different metals with stainless steel instruments in an autoclave you will soon find that 'stainless' is a misnomer. However clean or sterile they may be they just won't look it to the patient. We will return to the subject of autoclaves shortly.

As a spin-off from instruments, do not forget the need for a good sturdy shoe horn, a foot sander (the Lispro foot sander is one of the best), and also the appropriate applicators for dressings like Tubegauze – preferably in metal rather than very breakable plastic!

In bygone days, chiropodists would use solid scalpels and sharpen them with a hone and a strop. Some chiropody kits may still contain such weapons. However, if your practice will be domiciliary only, forget them. By all means use them for hobby work or cutting the carpet, but they do not belong in a visiting case.

For domiciliary work you can only really consider using disposable blades. These come pre-sterilised by gamma radiation and are used on the basis of one per patient. It is good to have several handles, especially if you are likely to use more than one size of blade on a given patient. The most well-known handle size is number 3. Popular sizes of blades include number 15 (for general and detailed work), number 10 (for larger areas of callous), and number 11 (for enucleation of corns). There are some very tiny blades and chisels with their own special handles for very detailed work. Because these blades are far more expensive you may choose to sterilize and re-use them, but the general purpose blades should be used once only, then discarded. To keep things really simple it is possible to do almost everything with a number 15 blade. Since blades are for single use there is little point in spending extra on stainless steel blades. Pre-sterilized carbon steel blades are quite adequate.

Make a point of showing the patient that the blade used on them comes out of a sterile packet, and after use goes straight into a suitable container for disposal. This emphasises to the patient that you care and puts them at ease. The previous chiropodist may have been just as careful, but may not have made the patient aware of this. There are a number of different sharps containers on the market, which allow you to remove the blade from the handle safely without coming into contact with the sharp end. The blades can then be transferred into a proper yellow sharps bin for final disposal.

So how do you finally get rid of the things? Do not be tempted to put your collection of used blades out with the household rubbish. You will be breaking the law if you do. Household rubbish normally goes for landfill and there is always the slight chance that someone further down the line could be injured if you do this. Used sharps are hazardous waste and need to be incinerated.

Your local cleansing department will be able to advise you on disposal. There are commercial firms like Rentokil who undertake this work. Or, you may come to some arrangement with someone who already has a sharps collection service, like a local hospital, nursing home, or patient on dialysis or insulin injections. It is a sad reflection on our times that yellow sharps containers are now provided in the toilet areas of some motorway services for public use. So there really is no excuse for not disposing of used scalpel blades responsibly.

Sterilisation and disinfection

Disposable blades (and possibly disposable drill burrs) are one thing, but for all your main instruments you will need to have a clear policy for sterilisation and disinfection. At times there are government guidelines on cross infection, and your professional association should have issued specific guidelines for your use. Regulations, procedures and available equipment do change with time, so you ignore the latest thinking on the matter at your peril!

First it would be well to remember that sterilisation and disinfection are not two interchangeable words, although some writers use the former rather carelessly. Simply put, sterilisation removes *all* micro-organisms. Disinfection doesn't! As far as scientifically possible, sterilisation deals with absolutes. Something is either sterile or it isn't. To talk about something being nearly sterile or semi-sterile is a bit like saying that someone is nearly pregnant. You either are or you're not! So there can be no half measures in a genuine sterilisation policy.

Obviously, by comparison, disinfection is a lot easier to achieve. For procedures like skin preparation or cleaning work surfaces, disinfection is the best you can do. For chiropodial instruments it is not!

You need to have a policy to cover three separate situations faced each day in practice. First, what do you do before you leave home? Obviously this can compare with surgery practice. Second, what can you do when travelling from place to place? Third, the actual treatment of the individual patient. The real problem to address is that while instruments may be 'sterile' when removed from their steriliser, they can go from 'sterile' to just 'disinfected' in a very short time indeed. Unless you are very careful they will not even be that by the time they reach the patient's foot.

Over the years various methods have been tried, many involving the application of heat. The most basic was to boil your instruments in water, but this is now proven to not destroy all pathogens, while doing a good job of ruining the cutting edge of clippers and scalpels. If your practice is in the Amazonian rain forest and nothing else is available – well – needs must, but we can generally consign that one to history.

Then there is the use of chemicals, mainly featuring glutaraldehyde. With chemicals, disinfection can be achieved in a fairly short time, whereas sterilisation can take up to ten hours – which feels like for ever! And once achieved (assuming it really can be achieved successfully by this method) how do you maintain that in the journey from chemical bath to patient's foot? And once used, back they need to be dunked for a day before you can think of using 'sterile' tools again. For modern domiciliary chiropody – forget it.

Returning to the principle of heat, glass bead sterilisers were once the in-thing. A chamber containing a myriad of tiny glass beads is heated up to extreme temperature, and the tools are burrowed into the beads. While this may still have value as a back-up in a surgery, glass bead sterilisers are not exactly the flavour of the month when it comes to portability. True, they are small, but once used a myriad of red hot glass beads are best left where they are, rather than risk being scattered all over someone's carpet. And tools when extracted, handles and all, are going to be hot, hot, hot.

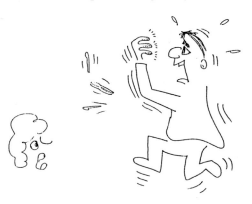

Objectively, at this time of writing, there is only one method of sterilisation that meets current criteria (i.e. that is guaranteed to work) and is feasible for chiropodists with a small surgery or domiciliary practice. This is the steam autoclave providing very high temperature steam under controlled pressure.

Using an autoclave

While it is possible to take an autoclave with you on domiciliary visits – there are certain portable models looking rather like a toasted cheese sandwich maker – unless you are based at a central point in somewhere like a nursing home it can get very complicated. It can also take too long to wait for a cycle to finish before extracting hot and damp tools to use.

The only feasible way for domiciliary work is to not only purchase an autoclave, but also sufficient sets of instruments that can be sterilised before you venture forth each day, transported to various feet in sealed airtight containers.

You are probably thinking that this all sounds ominously expensive. Frankly, to start in safe practice – it is! However, an autoclave is far more important than a state of the art drill, or portable cryo equipment, or other specialised equipment you may want. Some of these other items you can manage without for now, and in some cases, you will continue to manage without. You cannot safely manage without proper sterilising procedures.

Since an autoclave must be 100% effective – or forget it – this is the one purchase to buy new with a guarantee and test certificate that gives you a full twelve months before it needs to be tested again. If you do buy second-hand, you need to make sure that the model is up to the latest regulations, and want a test certificate with it dated last week. Failing that you should get it tested by a qualified person who can give you a valid certificate before you use it. All this extra hassle and expense will still make buying new the best long-term option.

While we are spending money like there's no to-morrow, you might want to add an ultrasound cleaner to the shopping list as well. It is vital before any tool is sterilised that the instrument is CLEAN. You might soak them for a while to allow loose debris to float off. You might also scrub them under hot running water with a dash of detergent using a stiff nail brush or smoker's toothbrush, but remember that *they* must be cleaned afterwards as well. Certain instruments like Black's files can easily retain organic matter if you are not very careful. If your autoclave bakes that on – as it surely will – your procedures have been a waste of time. Note for instance that the Hepititis B virus has been known to survive in a tiny speck of dried blood for up to six months. It cannot be stressed enough, before attempting to sterilise your instruments they MUST BE CLEAN.

So while an ultrasound cleaner can be yet more expense, you may soon find that the time saved, and the confidence engendered, make it a worthwhile investment. Tap water and a small amount of special detergent are placed in the vessel, the instruments are placed in a wire basket and lowered in, and for a few minutes ultrasound waves act as an invisible scrubbing brush, reaching the parts that other cleaners can't reach. It is quite a fascinating procedure to watch. It can also be quite sobering to see how much debris can be dislodged from instruments that, to the naked eye, looked clean!

Then take them out, rinse and dry them, and they are ready for the autoclave.

The simplest steam autoclaves (and the cheapest) look very much like what they really are — a fancy pressure cooker. (In some parts of the world it has not been unknown for a pressure cooker to be called into service as an emergency measure, although I wouldn't fancy the next casserole that came out of it!)

They have a set of very simple, idiot-proof, controls. These amount to filling the chamber to a specified mark with distilled water (obtainable from most garages), filling an internal bucket with tools, putting the lid on properly, and pressing one button. Lighted panels then tell you when the cycle is complete.

You can buy special instrument cassettes to use inside your autoclave, which are then taken along to the patient and opened in their presence. However, these do come expensive and mean that you have to obtain a full set of instruments for each patient. They also don't last for ever, so can continue to be expensive. It is a matter of personal preference, but a much cheaper option is to use self-seal sterilisation pouches or envelopes (commonly called 'steribags') made of special plastic and paper. Bought in bulk they are very cheap, and individual tools can be transported in them. While you will need standard clippers and a file for most patients, not everyone is going to need your ingrown nippers, or Blacks file, or probe, or drill burr, so you can manage with far fewer of these and only open the appropriate steribags as required.

While you can transfer the sterilised instruments from the autoclave and into bags and seal them after sterilisation, this is not ideal, as they are exposed to the atmosphere as well as handled for that short time.

(You can always wear sterile gloves or use sterile tongs for this, but how complicated do you want life to be?) It will be safer and a lot less trouble to place the tools in the bag, seal them down, and then put the sealed bag in the autoclave. Although the bags are partly made of paper – this is to allow the steam through – they will not disintegrate as long as they are treated carefully. Just watch any sharp points and spring mechanisms on some clippers as you insert them in the bags. Most brands of steribag have a strip of paper you can place inside which changes colour to show that sterilisation has been achieved, which can be a great comfort! The biggest problem is that, unless your autoclave has a drying cycle, which it probably will not, the bags will come out damp. Getting them dry all adds to the preparation time. So while it is possible to come home part way through a day and sterilise your tools for the afternoon shift, you will soon find it more practical to build up your supply of instruments so you really can sally forth at the start of a working day with sufficient in hand. Allowing for drying time it is easiest to do your autoclaving the night before.

Having gone to all the trouble of taking sterile tools to a patient, don't then blow it all by sloppy practice. Once your instruments are out of their steribags, be very careful where you put them. Consider using a disinfection spray on them between moves, and at times, the need to open a new bag for a replacement item if something nasty has been encountered and treated. Once used, place them back in the opened bags and then in a special container to take home. A large red pencil case can nicely look the part.

To the extent that you have control in someone else's home, keep your working environment clean. Your case, which in many instances may double as your work surface, must be clean. It can collect unwanted debris from patients all too easily, so it needs to be cleaned thoroughly for each trip. Everything you use should be kept within the clean environment of your case and thus isolated as much as possible from their surroundings. If you use any table of the patient's, at the very least cover it with a disposable paper towel that you supply.

And finally, whatever you do, keep all pets out of the room! No matter how impassioned are testimonials of unswerving obedience for assorted cats, dogs, and feathered friends – do not believe them! One cold nose of Fido in your case and you are in serious trouble. Impress

on owners that the experience could seriously damage Fido's health —
that will get compliance if nothing else will!

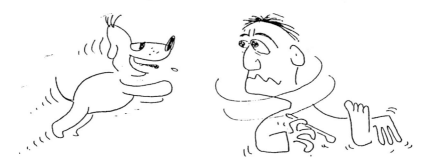

All the extra time and expense that correct aseptic procedures take
should be explained simply to the new patient. They should understand
that your fees don't just cover those minutes with their feet, but all the
preparation time, equipment costs and expertise for their safety that is
built into their treatment. If any local competitor is still out there
slicing away with one set of tools — be it from a jar of disinfectant
slopping about in the car, or worse, straight from the case — patients
will quickly understand why you charge what you do. Most will pay to
be safe rather than sorry. Wouldn't you?

A final warning

For basic chiropody some may feel that the above preoccupation with
autoclaving is all a bit over the top. It may even be argued that
chiropody has a good record and the risks of serious disease
transmission is very small. Whatever the odds, whatever the history,
you have a legal and moral obligation to do the very best you can for
the comfort and safety of your patient. Any potential or practising
chiropodist who does *not* have an autoclave should serious consider
some 'IFs':

- IF your patient developed an infection after your treatment (or
  any already existing condition flared up) could you *prove* you
  were not part of the problem if you had not used an autoclave?

- IF you were unable to do that, would your professional association still support you in any legal action against you?

- IF your association distanced itself from you, would your insurers still support you in any claim against you?

- IF there is any remote possibility of your insurers' ever dumping you because you have ignored clear practice guidelines, what protection do you personally have to practise chiropody? What protection do your patients have?

There is your worse case scenario. If you don't already have an autoclave – get one! Do it now!

Padding and strapping

You have limited space in you case, and your aim with its contents as always should be to keep things simple.

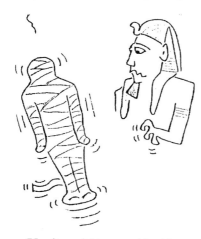

'He always did have trouble with metatarsal strapping ...'

It is possible to do almost everything with just a very few basics, especially since padding materials can be doubled up for extra thickness if required. Although only a small percentage of the population are allergic to plaster, it is simpler to get hypoallergenic types as a matter of course for all patients.

A minimum suggested list would be as follows:

Fleecy web. This can be used to prevent sheering stress and make very thin pads, crescents, rings, etc. Because it stretches, as long as you get the stretch in the right direction you can go round corners and over bumps and have a very neat result.

5 mm semi-compressed felt. This is for when thicker padding is required, e.g. hallux valgus crescents, metatarsal and other plantar pads.

Foam tubing. There are a variety of 'appliances' you can make with foam tubing (trade names include Tubifoam, Foamband, Protectofoam) if soft padding is required. These include toe separators, toe props, corn protectors, bunion shields and removable metatarsal pads. Those that prove successful for any particular patient can be reinforced with other strapping or covering materials and will then last a lot longer.

2.5 cm and 5 cm conforming adhesive strapping. These very thin dressings (trade names include Mefix, Fixomull Stretch, Chirofix) are ideal, because as with fleecy web, you can travel neatly over irregular terrain, and also overlap to produce a very satisfactory result, which lasts! (Some times to your horror the patient can allow it to last for several months between appointments!) The 5 cm size is ideal because you have sufficient width to cut a variety of shapes, and can peel the backing paper away from the centre without spoiling the edges.

Rigid strapping. There are rare occasions where the stretchy nature of the above is contra-indicated, where correction rather than just 'retention' is required. For example, the patient may have a painful nail sulcus, so a more rigid strapping can be affixed about an eighth of an inch from the offending edge, and the flesh pulled away as the strapping is anchored around the toe. This can bring immediate relief, and also allow you more room to work on the problem. When starting in practice, rigid strapping can give you the 'third hand' you may feel you need, although as you gain experience you will learn to manage without.

Tubegauze. This is ideal for keeping dressings in place on toes, particularly those on the apex. If ever you need just a gauze square it can be easily cut from a tubegauze roll. Because it stretches in all directions the 01 size will suit most toes. It can also be used to make anchorage loops on removable appliances, although elastic stockinette would normally last longer.

Micropore. This very thin tape is very well-known as being hypo-allergenic and some patients will specially ask for it. It is so well known and respected by the general public there is good sense in giving them what they want.

Cotton wool. For general cleansing and to manage all those runny items considered under 'materia medica' you will need good old-fashioned cotton wool. Gauze squares can be used as an alternative, but cotton wool comes cheaper. You can get a great quantity of cotton wool balls very cheaply indeed.

Materia medica

The limits of your chosen field of practice will determine what you actually need in the way of medicaments, and a lot will come down to what you as an individual get on well with, but again our concern should always be to keep things as simple as possible.

To cover the various aseptic procedures there are a wide variety of commercial preparations available from chiropody suppliers. They will tell you which current ones are suitable for skin preparation prior to surgery, or for ongoing disinfection of instruments once released from their steribag protection. They come in containers of various shapes and sizes, including ozone-friendly aerosols, so available space in your case can influence your choice. However, it is always good psychology to additionally have with you a well-known and well-respected mild antiseptic as a liquid or cream. A mysterious fluid out of a dropper bottle is one thing, but for general use a familiar tube or familiar packaging helps put patients at ease.

One antiseptic you will want to carry is hydrogen peroxide (10 volumes solution). This presents a quite spectacular bubbling action if there is any infection present, and is ideal for shifting debris out of cavities in these circumstances. One very practical use too is in treating the familiar D-I-Y version of an ingrown nail. You often have great difficulty in seeing the offending splinter the patient's own mangling has left because of the swelling. Attempts to use a probe directly send the patient through the roof and you only have to look at it and it bleeds! Sometimes you can very gently insert a small piece of cotton wool down the side of the nail with a probe. You then add a couple of drops of hydrogen peroxide. After a short interval while you treat something else, the cotton wool can be eased out, and the effects of the hydrogen peroxide will have created a gap where you can now at least see the problem, and without hurting the patient.

Tincture benzoin co. (Friar's Balsam) is also mildly antiseptic, and has a variety of uses. If a patient is allergic to plaster, or if there are difficulties getting ordinary dressings to stay on, a coating of Friar's balsam is of great assistance. For masking areas of skin in treating verrucae, for keeping nail packing in place, or for anchoring wobbly soft corns for surgery, it has its value. All in all tinct. benzoin co. is very versatile. The biggest problem is that it is also very messy. Get it on someone's clothes or carpet and you have got problems! You can get good control by using it from a dropper bottle, although you may have trouble getting the top off after a while.

Unlike the 'last chiropodist' *you* never make anyone bleed – you hope – . . . Well, it can happen to the best. So you need to carry a styptic of some sort with you., even if just an alum stick or silver nitrate pencil.

There are some contra-indications with styptics (see section THE VISIT) so this must be taken on board. Silver nitrate pencil can also be used as a diagnostic for verrucae, and for treating vascular corns, and lower strengths can be used as an astringent or to complete corn removal.

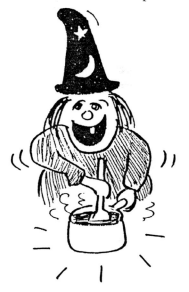

You will want to carry with you some of the commercial preparations from the suppliers for tinea pedis and fungal problems of the nails. Remember the maxim that for success the preparations should be used for at least a month after the problem appears to have gone away. If you are treating verrucae by chemical means then you will need the popular 60% strength of salicylic acid or a preparation of your choice. Out of the standard 'off the shelf' preparations for verrucae, this writer has found the greatest success with 'Glutarol' – but the trouble with verrucae is that every chiropodist will tell you something different!

For finishing off nails after drill work, or to hold nail packing in place (as an alternative to messy tinct. benz.) Acrytensil is a good stand-by.

Then there are silicones for corrective or palliative devices. Otoform-K, which was originally developed for making individual hearing aids, is a good economical starter. Many practitioners stay with it. Then there are the foot creams – an industry all by itself. There are creams with exotic names for every imaginable kind of skin and skin condition, but for general use E-45 has proved its worth. With some creams you may be paying double the price for what amounts to a bit of perfume. You must decide, but simple E-45 has a lot going for it.

Looking the part

The final piece of equipment to consider is what we actually wear. Here reasonableness should prevail. You may have some unpleasant places to visit, but you are not with a decontamination unit visiting Chernobyl, you are simply a visiting chiropodist. To look the part the main thing you need to wear is a white coat or jacket. To save continually changing throughout the day you may want it on all the time, but then wear a discreet coat on top in the street – depending on the weather. Walking down the road in a white coat can be

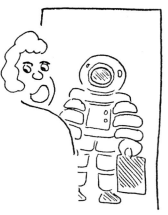

'It's the chiropodist!'

impressive, but it can also appear pretentious, and make the neighbours wonder what on earth you are doing. (What you *are* doing is collecting a lot of street dust and dirt on your white coat and taking it into close contact with the patient!)

Make sure that your coat stays white by having at least two, so that one is always fresh from the wash. Cuffs can look grubby very quickly, particularly if you neglect to roll up your sleeves properly when washing your hands. Although cotton is more expensive than polyester it can be boiled and bleached and so stay presentable longer – as long as someone else does the ironing!

What about gloves, masks, eyeshields..? (theatre wear, suit of armour, space helmet?)

Wearing latex gloves is becoming more common. Some chiropodists swear by them, others at them. By all means try them; it can look very impressive, but you may settle for the full mobility of properly cleansed hands. However, if you do not use gloves the patient will be observing your hands very closely if they take any interest in what you are doing. Make sure that your finger nails are short and manicured, and that evidence of working on the car last night is not present! If you wear gloves remember that they provide little protection against a sharps injury!

You may want to carry a supply of disposable paper masks with you for drill work. If you do not normally wear glasses you may consider eye-shields. However, you can minimise the danger of nail splinters in your eye (or up your nose) by placing the thumb carefully over the nail when doing nail trims. This will contain any unidentified flying objects.

Handling Patients

The telephone

The telephone is your lifeline. Unless you have a friend or relative who can sit by the telephone for twenty-four hours a day (and who sounds like a receptionist!) a good answerphone is also essential. For collecting a number of messages, a machine with two tapes is more efficient. (One tape contains your outgoing message and the other records the incoming calls.) Single tape machines, if collecting a number of messages, have a habit of leaving people listening to a long collection of bleeps. They are then more likely to get nervous or angry (some people have a pathological hatred of answerphones) and put the phone down. Some machines only allow for a very brief incoming message, and callers easily run out of time before giving you the two essentials you need – their name and telephone number.

With an answerphone you can announce a twenty-four hour answering service and leave it on all night. When fed up with callers you can turn it on while you settle down to watch the news ...

Your own announcement must be clear and professional. Do not be tempted by cassettes offering impersonations of Mickey Mouse and Prince Charles! If necessary, write something down and practice it until it sounds right. A suitable message could be: *'This is a recorded message – John Smith the chiropodist speaking. I am sorry I am not available to answer your call personally, but if you would like to leave your NAME and TELEPHONE NUMBER I will call you back as soon as possible. If you would like to leave a message you have as long as you like to do so after you hear the tone. Thank you for calling'.*

If your machine only allows them 30 seconds recording time, then tell them that in your message and stress NAME and TELEPHONE NUMBER only. If you go away on holiday or close for a few days, a message must tell callers this, and that you will call them back after a stated date. Otherwise you may get a collection of messages from the same person with increasing concern or annoyance that they have not heard from you.

What about those who put the telephone down and will not leave a message? Without an Ansaphone you would have lost them anyway. Most people if told clearly that all you need is a name and number will pluck up courage and leave that – even if they have to telephone again to do so. It is the ones who start talking and then wish they hadn't and don't quite know how to stop that make for the most entertaining listening on playback. But don't tell them that!

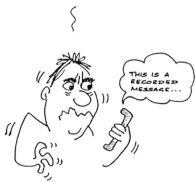

Mobile phones

Everything you can do with a land line and more can also be done with the omnipresent mobile phone. The average family appears to have 2.4 of them – and the figure is rising. However, unless you enjoy being interrupted in chiropodial mid-slice, or wish to be another statistic as with phone clamped to an ear you veer across the highway, you will not want the thing turned on for most of the day. Where the mobile scores is the ability to rescue messages from its Ansaphone service while out in practice. On occasion this may give you greater flexibility in slotting in patients when already in their area. In a rural practice this can be of help. On the downside, making appointments on the hoof can only work effectively if you are prepared to carry all your patient records around with you, in a box, or on a laptop, on the off-chance you might need them. On reflection, you may well settle for catching your calls at the end of the day, when you can quietly and calmly plan future appointments to suit your movements.

Perhaps the best use of the mobile, apart from handling breakdowns or radioing home for supplies (tea, coffee, brandy, etc.) is the not-at-home scenario. You have arrived at a patient's home, whose doorbell does not work and whose new PVC door is impervious to the sound of a hammering fist, and whose occupant is aurally impaired. What do you do as the wind and rain lash down on you, your case and the doorstep? You phone them up, that's what you do!

When returning calls you will have everything you need on hand. But make sure that when you answer the telephone personally you are also ready to handle enquiries. Assume at the outset that every time the telephone rings it is a new patient. As a matter of course have your appointments book and your record cards by the telephone. The prospective patients usually assume they are telephoning a surgery. They have a mental image of a clinical environment, people in white coats, receptionists, dog-eared motoring magazines on the table, and so forth. Nothing will disillusion them sooner than the sounds of frantic rummaging, and muffled calls to other family members to find your appointments book!

After establishing that – yes – you are the chiropodist, and that the caller wishes to make an appointment and is not just asking for advice, there are certain points you need to briefly cover while you make notes:

1. 'Have I seen you before?' It may feel a little strange saying this for the first two months in practice, but it is a good habit to get into. If you have, then you need their record card from the file and can very easily make an appointment. If they are new patients then explain that you will need to take just a few details.

2. Unless they ask 'Do you make home visits?' explain the nature of your practice at the outset – you will go to them rather than have them come to you. There are some people who will really want a surgery. If that is the case, don't try and talk them into something they don't want! You are not a double glazing salesman! Explain that if they have a problem getting an appointment at a surgery and want to come back to you that will be quite all right. If necessary, refer them to a surgery you can recommend.

3. With a new patient, ask briefly what the problem is. Establish that this is something you can treat. If it is outside your field, then find that out now. The patient will not thank you for turning up ten days later and then saying sorry... On rare occasions you will establish that the person's first visit should be to the doctor or even the casualty department at the local hospital!

If the problem involves sepsis, advice on saline footbaths can be given, or in some cases you may refer them to the doctor for a course of antibiotics before you can effectively treat them. If you have decided not to treat verrucae on domiciliary visits, and that is what they believe they have, explain the benefits of a surgery and refer them. Of course patients have mistakenly called all manner of callosities verrucae, so a little probing is helpful. Have they tried the layman's test for verrucae? If they press down on the area does it hurt? (Likely not.) If they squeeze across it does it hurt? (Very likely so!) If there is doubt, explain that you cannot diagnose very easily over the telephone, but you are prepared to come and see them and advise them. If they are happy with that, then all well and good.

If the problem is within your field of practice, but requires more specialist equipment, finding out over the telephone ensures you take whatever is needed with you.

4. You will take a proper medical history when you see the patient in person, but with a new enquiry – are they diabetic? If yes, is their management by diet, tablets or injections? If you cannot see them for several days and something sounds wrong, then it is urgent they seek professional advice immediately. If you have only recently started out in practice and would rather refer the chronic diabetic to a proper surgery or diabetic clinic, then now at the telephone stage is the time to do it.

5. 'When did you last have chiropody treatment?' You may choose to save this until you see them personally, but it is an important question. If the answer is never, they may well need some reassurance as to what is involved. If it was two weeks ago, why do they want to see you, and who did they see last time? Your ethical code and other factors may well ring warning bells with this patient.

6. I knew of one chiropodist who once conducted such a telephone inquisition, put the phone down, and then found himself looking at a date, time and name – but no address or telephone number... So after all the above, do not forget those essentials, along with brief directions to find their address if necessary. Be prepared for

the fact that a large number of the population literally do not know their left from their right when giving directions! Note their telephone number, just in case you have to rearrange their appointment or contact them for any reason.

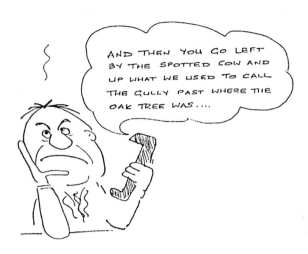

7. Conclude by telling them they have 'passed the audition' and make sure *they* have a clear grasp of the date and approximate time of your visit. Impress on them that you cannot be 100% precise on the time, because of factors like traffic conditions, and the time the previous patient may require, but normally you would be within say twenty minutes either way of the appointment time. Please could they be ready for you.

It may sound a lot, but in practice can be accomplished very quickly in a pleasant but efficient manner, and you can then make the house call knowing reasonably well what to expect.

The visit

On arrival at the patient's home there are several things you will need to organise before you start.

First, you will need to be able to wash and dry your hands, both before and after treatment. Before, because you are not bringing anything nasty with you, and after, because you have no intention of taking anything nasty away with you! Depending on the type of household you can use their soap and towel, or supply your own, in which case a special antibacterial preparation would be in order.

You will then need the patient to supply you with an additional towel for the treatment itself. Unless it suits your style to use a foot rest or tray when operating, the patient's foot can rest on your knees on top of their own towel, to which ideally you add a small paper one. At the end of the treatment you carefully fold in the paper towel ('to see that no bits go on the carpet') and hand it over for disposal ('here are a few bits of your foot as a souvenir...'). With elderly patients who live alone you may need to dispose of the contents for them in the rubbish bin. On occasion you may need to take soiled dressings away with you in sealed polythene bags for proper disposal. The one piece of rubbish you must *never* leave behind is disposable scalpel blades. (See STERILISATION for sharps disposal.)

If you will be using a drill that requires mains electricity, you will need access to a power point. With a new patient it is best to plug in at the outset. Chiro's law states that if you do not plug it in – you will be

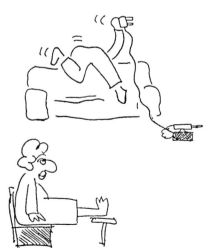

bound to need it! Unless the householder has difficulties it is better to let them plug it in for you.

People seem to have power points hidden in the most awkward places, behind ton weight settees, for instance, or to have spaghetti junction connections into the sockets. If someone is going to mess up the video or turn off the freezer, let it be them not you! Again of course with elderly or immobile patients you may need to help them, but do check carefully what you can and cannot pull out of the sockets.

You then need something to sit on! If you have a bad back it is worth considering a portable fold-up operator's stool or chair, so that you are always at a height you can cope with, but of course this is more lumber to carry around. In most homes it is possible to improvise with a stool or chair, as long as you are not higher than the patient when seated. Beware the D.I.Y. square 'pouffe' that looks as light as a feather, but when you try and lift it appears to be filled with bricks (usually old catalogues)!

You will have already obtained certain information over the telephone and should have a partially completed record card with you. Now you are set up there are still a few more details you will need.

You need the name of their doctor. You may need to refer the patient or write a letter to their doctor. It is surprising how many people do not know the name of their doctor or doctors, but you will soon come to know the various practices in your area. It builds confidence in the new patient when you know the proper name of their G.P. when they often don't.

Then you need a medical history from them. Are they having any medicines? You need to know what they are on and why. A little tactful probing is necessary. Patients are quite capable of saying they don't take any medicines, and then spring it on you later that they only take tablets... So you need to spell it out: are they taking anything from the chemist or prescribed by the doctor?

You are not expected to be a pharmacist and know every drug in common usage along with its contra-indications. So it is useful to carry with you a copy of M.I.M.S. or one of the commercially produced books such as 'Medicines – A Comprehensive Guide' published very cheaply by Paragon. Take time to check tablets, and you will soon come to know the common ones for blood pressure, circulatory problems, water retention, etc. if you did not know them already.

If they are on blood thinners like Warfarin this immediately gives a red warning light! It would be wrong to say 'take special care' because really you should take special care with everyone. But the last thing you want to do is make this particular patient bleed. So you may need to be extra conservative in the extent of the treatment you give, and explain why.

In the unhappy event that there is a slight haemorrhage, styptics that induce clotting are not advised. This person is not on anti-clotting agents for fun; your styptic could just possibly not be good for them! So elevation, application of cotton wool (or better still a product like Kaltostat), pressure and patience is the answer. In difficult cases the medical profession may take the patient off Warfarin or equivalent for a few days until healing is established, but you are there to help the patient, not give them something else to worry about! So be alert to the danger signals such as anti-coagulants or the suggestion of diabetes, remembering that not all patients know or admit their true situation. Know how far you can safely use your scalpel with any specific patient, and when it is wise to stop.

Taking such a case history will have been dealt with in your basic training, but always remember that nothing remains constant. As we age, more things tend to go wrong with us; so do check each time that there is no new medication being taken or relevant condition being treated by others.

Once you have completed this part of the paperwork you can make a detailed examination of the foot, and mark on your chart what requires attention. This will be your permanent record for future visits. Do not do anything until after you have examined carefully and made notes on both feet. There is nothing worse for an inexperienced chiropodist to start work on what appears to be the main problem, and then find when running out of time that this was the patient's 'good foot'. If time is limited and the person has come to you after years of neglect, they may need more than one appointment. By examining both feet in detail before you do anything you can decide what has to be done in the time allocated for the first visit.

If the patient has never had chiropody treatment before or has had a bad experience in the past, they will need some reassurance. With the nervous patient hold the foot firmly (but not too tight) and talk to them! In my practice area people are naturally gregarious. They are nosey and like to know your business. Turning it back on them – 'Where are you from? How long have you lived here?' – usually opens the floodgates. While they talk away, their mind is off what you are doing, which with good technique should normally be painless anyway.

Some people are scared stiff at the sight of the drill, with horrible memories of the last visit to the dentist. So reassure them: it is not like the dentist at all, it is just like a motorised pumice stone. Do *not* say that

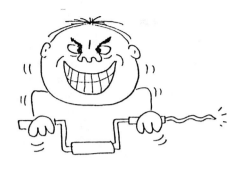

if all else fails you'll get out the Black and Decker... Explain that the only thing that might happen with the drill is that it can get a bit warm. However, if anything does not feel right they must let you know ("Because I can't look at your feet and your face at the same time") and you will stop immediately.

If there are special requirements that would be useful to know in advance next time, make sure you note these down, e.g. silicones needed, allergic to plaster, drill not required, insists on Micropore, extra time needed. The patient will not remind you the next time they telephone, and you will not remember without the notes on the card.

Throughout an appointment you will have a certain set routine to follow. As well as all the preliminary writing, keep good records of what you do to the patient, and why. The bottom line with a patient's card is – what would your insurers require if ever there were a dispute or attempted claim against you?

At the end of your treatment make sure the patient is happy before you leave. If they are mobile make them give their feet 'a test run'. If there are instructions about their shoes, or wearing a silicone appliance the right way up – make sure they understand. Do not be in too much of a hurry to rush away. Half an hour after you have gone you still want them to be enthusing how good you were!

Patient care and conversation

There is an old adage for medical practitioners: do not make friends of your patients, or patients of your friends. From the patient's side of the counter this reads: don't go to a friend – go to someone you can sue!

There must be a certain amount of reserve or professional detachment. People expect that. They respect it. They do not respect over-familiarity, and can easily change to another chiropodist whose slightly distant manner makes them feel more comfortable and safe.

Having made that point, remember that a number of your patients may be elderly or housebound. In these instances you could be their only visitor of the day or even week. So you do need the art of conversation.

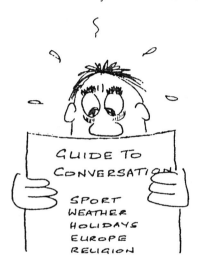

More than talking this often means being a good listener. Do not expect to be allowed to rush through your treatment and escape! Be prepared for the family history. Be prepared for the offer of umpteen cups of tea or coffee, and have strategies for appreciative refusal – unless you want to be searching for the loo on too many occasions during the day. Many of the housebound will have previously had NHS domiciliary treatment, and it is the appearance of haste, as the chiropodist tries to visit a lot of people in a very short time that has made them decide to 'go private'. So in a sense they are paying for your time and attention, as well as their treatment. Give them what they want, within reason, and you are fulfilling a valuable function. They will be happy, and will want you back on a regular basis.

So what do you talk about with patients? As discussed under THE VISIT some useful openings are – Where are you from? Have you always lived here? Add – Are these your grandchildren in this photograph? – and you are away! It is a rare patient who will flatly tell you to mind your own business, but if any make it clear they do not want conversation then that must be respected. There are of course traditional subjects that most will still view as taboo, like politics and religion. But you will find some people who will ignore these conventions and have very fixed views on certain things. There is a real art in being pleasantly non-committal on a wide variety of topics! If you personally have very firm views on any matter just take care. There is a time and a place for everything. This time and this place is for footcare – not a heated debate on the economy or a re-run of the reformation! If you choose to 'do battle' do not be surprised if the patient decides for a less tiring treatment from someone else next time.

One very important point in conversation – do *not* run down other chiropodists! It is totally unprofessional! If you have any partisan feelings about your own professional association, keep them to yourself! If the patient volunteers a horror story about a previous experience, be generally understanding, but remember you are only hearing one side. If it is a NHS domiciliary visit that was too brief, or is three months overdue, be aware of the current financial constraints on the service in your area. Be aware too of how patients can obtain NHS treatment locally. If they really cannot afford your fees then it would be a kindness to direct them accurately to what is available.

On the subject of NHS chiropody, you may get some unusual complaints at times. They say that it is a sign of old age when all the policemen start to look young. To many elderly, the NHS chiropodists look young – very young! Most who trained for State Registration come from schools and colleges. So on balance they are often younger than many trained in the private sector, who often come into chiropody after previous careers, for example in nursing. But some elderly patients get quite stroppy at the thought of visits from 'young girls' who they assume are 'still training' and who are 'not qualified' yet! They get even more stroppy when 'young girls' start families and leave the scene for a while, and are not always replaced. By all means be sympathetic in such a scenario, but be honest! Never over indulge a patient's misconceptions. For one thing, someone else may put them right, and where would that leave you? So make it clear that those in the public sector are 'proper chiropodists' and well qualified. As for skills in handling people and genuine feelings for people, then each practitioner must be judged as an individual.

With elderly patients who live on their own it is important to have details of their family, particularly if they live nearby. There may be occasions when you need to advise them that something needs attention. It could be a sudden increase in water retention when an old person forgets their diuretics, or evidence of a fall or some injury. You will naturally have details of their doctor to contact if necessary, but one of the first stops in less urgent matters is the family if they are supportive. You may advise someone to follow a course of treatment which they appear capable of handling, but you wonder if they will really do what you ask? If they will, for how long? Here again it is good to advise the relatives, or some other regular caller who can check and perhaps 'encourage them' between visits, so that it happens. There is obviously more scope if an elderly patient has relatives living with them. Showing someone else in the family which way up and on which foot your silicone device should go can make a great difference in its effectiveness between visits!

Broken appointments

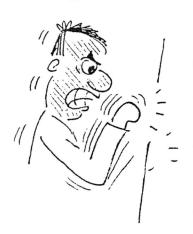

So you have motored all the way out to this desolate farm house, have travelled what seem like miles over muddy terrain that has destroyed the effects of yesterday's car wash, and now when you circumnavigate a yard full of cow pats and hammer on the door – THIS little piggy has gone to market... or somewhere... What do you do?

Fortunately in domiciliary work, the broken appointment does not happen very often. These people *want* to see you! Many will have been waiting indoors patiently all morning to be certain of seeing you. As long as you have not given an unrealistic expectation that you will be there exactly on the dot – so they can arrive home one minute before that – most patients will be there in good time and will wait if you are later than expected.

But it does happen sometimes. At the very least you need to show that you have called, either by putting a business card with a note on it through the letterbox, or if you are really well organised, using a specially produced slip for the occasion. If you do not care whether you ever do see them again or not, ask them to telephone you. (In

46

embarrassment some will then telephone another chiropodist instead.) If you want to see them again, you telephone them. If you are a hard-nosed professional then you will make a charge for the broken appointment, and your stationery, visiting and appointment cards will all carry the dire warnings to that effect. If you are soft, and it is a little old lady who got all muddled and thought it was next Tuesday, not this Thursday, and where was that appointment card you left me? – then you may let her off, the first time anyway.

If there is any danger with certain patients that they are going to forget the appointment – particularly when it has been made at the previous visit some weeks before – it can be very practical to operate a reminder system. You mark their card with a suitable sign – a red dot or a line with a colour marker – and as long as you organise each day's cards the night before, then you can telephone them and remind them you are coming. The cost of the telephone call can then be included in your professional fee for this patient.

Personal safety

There are some strange people out there. The question is sometimes raised, "What if..." It must be conceded that there is always a slight risk of assault – however small – in any trade or profession which requires visiting the public sight unseen on a one to one basis.

We have to accept that it is not generally practical to take around with you a 'minder' in the guise of a 'domiciliary care assistant'. Domiciliary work is literally one to one in most cases. Chiropodists are probably less at risk than some other visitors. The white coat can be a certain protection, and many of our patients are elderly. They may have the will for mischief, but not much else! So a practitioner just has to be careful, and if anything does not seem to be right about the surroundings or about the patient, then – to coin a phrase from the Sunday papers of yesteryear – you 'make an excuse and leave'.

If you personally have taken to carrying a pocket alarm or personal security device of some sort in ordinary life, then that can still travel with you in your work. Of course you might reason that you have a case full of lethal equipment, but the profession does not really want to see the headline *"But I stabbed him with a STERILE blade," says*

Chiropodist... You just have to take reasonable care. But quite frankly, if you are *that* anxious about what might just happen every time you are called out on a new patient, then domiciliary work is really not for you. It would be far better, and far less stressful in your case, to work from a surgery, where you can likely have someone else on hand.

If ever you do face the situation where you choose to leave because of the patient's misbehaviour, or if there is any danger they may make some sort of accusation against you, then you must make a detailed written report on the circumstances as soon as possible after you leave. Then you must decide how serious the matter really is, and just who now needs to see that report.

Practice Management

Obtaining patients

It may be a dirty word to some people, but initially the only way to obtain patients is to ADVERTISE. Some way or another the public has to learn that you exist and that you are available.

The Office of Fair Trading as good as removed advertising restrictions for chiropodists in 1987. However, you may still be limited to some degree by your professional association. Even if not, you certainly should remember the dignity of your profession in the ways that you get known.

Before reviewing the main ways of effectively doing this, a word of warning. Once you *are* known, you are quite likely to be approached by advertising salesmen, who offer you premium space in a new 'directory' or on a bulletin board at a health centre or hospital. If you contemplate going down either road, a few questions are in order. What area will a new directory cover? How many people will actually see it? Is it just going to be those who have been foolish enough to buy space in it? If you are offered space on a bulletin board or advertising board, where will it be located? Some new chiropodists have spent large sums of money on this kind of display advertising that has ended up behind a broom cupboard – or as near that fate as makes no difference! Ask yourself, when was the last time *I* looked at the small print on any hospital bulletin board?

It is your choice. It is your money. But there are several more reliable ways of obtaining patients. In this section we will consider personal recommendation, Yellow Pages and newspaper advertising, suitable places to leave business cards including nursing homes, lecturing to local groups, and some thoughts on professional fees.

Personal recommendations

With personal recommendation your patients do the advertising. It goes without saying that you have to be recommendable! In any sphere of life it can take years to build up a good reputation and about two minutes to lose it! So you must be good! People expect standards of hygiene, treatment, professional manners and a feeling that they, the patient, come first.

If you do not succeed here, then quite frankly you had better forget being a chiropodist and do something else! But if your patients are happy they will tell their friends. (If they are unhappy, they will also tell their friends!)

Long term, personal recommendation is probably the best way to build a practice. It is certainly the most satisfying. But it takes time. Usually it is slow starting, before a snowball effect takes over. That is why many full-time chiropodists started life as part-timers – or full-timers who sat around a lot! So you need time, and you also need some existing patients who are prepared to recommend you. This calls for more direct advertising.

Yellow Pages

The Yellow Pages directories cover the whole country, and Thompson's directories also cover many areas. Respected publications like these are the first place most people will look to find any local service they need. You need to get in them as soon as possible!

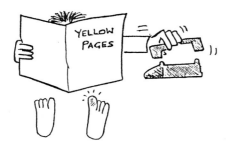

If you have a private telephone line to begin with, and are therefore not eligible for a free Yellow Pages entry, pay to go in! The cost may seem high, but unless you have a lot of time to build up the practice, it is essential.

The first year I entered Yellow Pages, I asked each new patient who telephoned how had they heard about me? Within less than three weeks of publication, the entry had more than paid for itself.

Newspaper advertising

The difficulty with newspaper advertising is that chiropodists always get lumped into the Personal columns ('shy attractive divorcee wishes to meet...') or worse still, under Personal Services ('...sent discreetly under plain wrappers'). It can also be very expensive, although rates in the plethora of 'free papers' are often cheaper than actual local newspapers. But they all have the disadvantage of being thrown out with tomorrow's potato peelings!

A small ad running for several weeks will soon cost more than Yellow Pages, which runs all year, and where far more people will look. From personal experience, save your money! If other local chiropodists are advertising there, do not worry. They are likely wasting theirs!

Of greater value can be gaining publicity through a news story or reader's letter. As long as it is not of the 'local chiropodist fined' variety, most publicity is good publicity! Attended a seminar? Foot Health week? Shortage of NHS services? Manning a first aid station in the local marathon? Tinea pedis epidemic? Gained an extra qualification? Write to the local rag about it!

Business cards

Before discussing where you can leave your business cards, a word about the business card itself. It is very important that you business cards *look* professional. If you go just for cheapness you may end up with a 'printer's job' – i.e. someone has printing equipment but no eye for design. So you end up with a mess, a mismatch of type faces which look what it is – cheap and nasty! It is good to check out other colleagues cards for ideas of design and recommendation of printers. Once you are certain you will not be changing your card, then get plenty. Costs drop dramatically for large orders.

On your card as well as the obvious professional details, the title *VISITING CHIROPODIST* or *VISITING CHIROPODY SERVICE* or *HOME VISITING SERVICE* says it all. If you want to appear upmarket your association's crest combined with *'HOME VISITS BY APPOINTMENT'* can look rather grand.

In circulating cards keep things low-key. In this country the public do not expect aggressive marketing by chiropodists. You are not selling cavity-wall insulation! Neither do people expect to see chiropody ads in the newsagent, or to have them dropping through the letter box like soap powder coupons. Professionally, this is not the way to win friends and influence people.

So where can you discreetly leave your card? Useful *people* to see include District Nurses, Home Help Supervisors, and also health care professionals or therapists in other fields. If your area has its share of physiotherapists, reflexologists, aromatherapists and the like – and if you personally can conscientiously recommend these people, then cards can be carried on a reciprocal basis.

Useful places to leave cards with permission include the chemists and shoe shops, OAP clubs, WI branches, and organisations like Age Concern.

A special mention must be made here of nursing homes and supermarkets and factories.

Nursing homes

As people live longer and families become more scattered and fragmented, nursing homes and retirement homes are one of the growth industries of the modern world.

Visit all the homes in your catchment area and leave your card. As with all 'advertising' your visit should be kept low-key, when 'passing through'. Do not be surprised if they already have a chiropodist – how would they have managed so far otherwise? So that's fine, but if ever they need to call *you* in, you are available and here is your card. If an existing patient moves into residential care, try and stick with them if you can and give them any 'nursing home reduction' in fee. It is well worth going to nursing homes for just the one resident. Unless they already have a first-class chiropodist in permanent attendance you will get known, and sooner or later it will grow. Once you have one or two homes on your books then these can be mentioned in passing to establish your bona fide status when visiting other establishments.

Nursing homes and retirement homes vary drastically in quality. Some homes run by the local council can be far superior in care and general atmosphere to expensive private operations. So much depends on the staff. But they can be very sad places, so – even if it is a bad day for you – try and be a ray of sunshine for the residents. If they welcome your visits (assuming of course they can remember them) then more residents will want you – not the next chiropodist who calls with his or her card.

If nursing home work is offered, it is good to get the rules outlined at the start. You are providing an essential service for them, generally because an overloaded state system cannot cope sufficiently in this area. To provide this service properly there are certain things you need from the home. For sterilisation purposes you may need a central point from which to work, and help from the care assistants to bring the patients to you and take them away again if they are not safely mobile. If you do not get this established at the outset, you risk being left on your own, travelling from room to room, struggling with heavy female patients whose 'stockings' invariably turn out to be 'tights'...

This may be more difficult to establish if you are first called in to see one patient on a private basis. This is not much different from seeing the patient in their own home; but once it becomes an official request to see a few more then establish the rules politely but clearly.

You may occasionally have difficulty in getting paid, unless you have talked arrangements through with the staff. The best arrangement of all is for the home to collect all the fees from the residents and then pay you on one cheque, for which they get your official receipt. In practice, some residents will want to pay you themselves, because they fiercely treasure this remaining bit of independence. Good communication between you and the senior staff is important, and receipts are essential. If the home pays for individuals out of their 'pocket money' they must have some official means of showing relatives where the money has gone.

Supermarkets and factories

Some chiropodists have had good success in canvassing the personnel managers of large stores or factories. Few firms today are prepared to financially subsidize their work force, but some will consider providing the medical or first aid room for your use, and allow workers a short time off work to come to you on a private basis. You have the luxury of a surgery (albeit limited) and the staff can get their chiropody treatment during working hours. A notice in the Ladies, or the staff notice board can advise them when your next visit will be.

In supermarkets and superstores be prepared for a changing float of patients, as many of these now only employ part-time staff on the shop floor. So the shift system pattern will dictate who is actually in work on the day you come.

Once you have the first store or factory, that can be quoted in passing when broadening your horizons, particularly if you approach others in the same market group.

Lectures

The local library will have details of local groups like the WI, WRVS, and the like. Those that arrange meetings are often desperate for speakers – so desperate they would even consider you! Of course if you

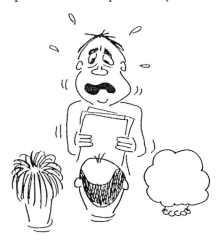

have a flare for that sort of thing, they will welcome you with open arms, and one invitation leads to another.

What can you talk about? Basic foot problems, basic anatomy of the foot, footwear and hosiery, self-help and when to see the chiropodist, etc. 20-30 minutes for a talk followed by a question and answer session will fill the time nicely. At the end you can leave your cards with those who want them.

The secret of speaking in these situations is to keep things very simple and basic, but with lots of humour. Someone else will have to write the Bumper Book of Chiropody Jokes, but do try and get them on your side quickly. One seasoned lecturer always starts: "If your feet hurt, you hurt..." (pause) and then inevitably comes the ragged chorus "...all over!" He then asks: "Why this is?" From then on the audience is with him.

In any question and answer session, as with personal conversations with patients, never run down other chiropodists. Be aware of the strengths and limitations of the local NHS chiropody service, but remember that you are not there either to defend or condemn it. However, you can certainly stress the benefits of private treatment, where the public can be treated when they want, where they want (i.e. at home), and by whom they want... (and if anyone would like to take a card...).

At the end of your lecture be prepared to then be asked to judge the flower arranging or sponge cake competition – by far the most fraught part of the evening!

If all the above is not your scene, but sounds like a potential nightmare, then forget it – but some chiropodists have generated much interest in this way. Even years later when people find they need treatment they will want to go to someone 'they know'.

Professional fees

Before concluding how to obtain patients, it is appropriate to consider what we charge them. Your professional fees must be realistic for your area, and for what you actually do! So you must fit into the general fee structure for your part of the world. This also affects your keeping patients, because a surprisingly large number are embarrassed to ask how much in advance, and only find out your charges after their first treatment.

If you are too expensive for your area, people will simply go elsewhere, unless you are more than very, very good. If you are too cheap, your expenditure will ultimately wipe out your living, you will annoy other practitioners, and in the long run people have a sixth sense that tells them that you get what you pay for!

You might consider making a reduction for OAP's within a certain radius of your home, or block reductions in places like nursing homes. But it is best to keep your fee structure as simple as possible. When someone telephones and this time asks: "How much?" you want to give them a figure, not – "It all depends..."

Rome was not built in a day. To build a successful domiciliary practice takes time. For patients – you need patience! Some private schools in their enthusiasm to train new chiropodists may tell success stories that are unrepresentative of your area. Do not be surprised if it takes a year or even longer to get established in secure full-time domiciliary chiropody. But once you are known, and have built a local reputation, you can be in a very secure profession.

There are, however, a number of things you can do to encourage your patients to come back to you, as the next section discusses.

Keeping patients

At the end of the line there is only one way to keep patients: to be good at your work!

Unless poor Joe Public is stuck with you because there is no alternative

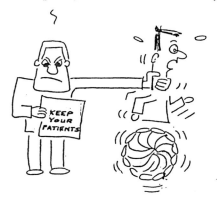

(an unlikely scenario) you have to be good! Yours may be a limited field, but within that field never cut corners or short-change your patients. So before anything else, work on that and never forget that!

So with that sermon out of the way, what can we do when there *is* a choice of practitioner, and we assume they are all good at what they do?

Once a patient has been treated by you they need to feel that *you* are now *their* chiropodist. If they are happy with your treatment this bond can be automatic. If they need regular maintenance then a proper cycle can start with a new appointment made at the end of each old one. But if they are the more casual patient with an occasional one-off problem, you want some way of reminding them that you are their chiropodist, and that periodic treatment would not be a bad idea.

We now look at five basic tools that can keep you – *THEIR CHIROPODIST* – as a ray of sunshine on the horizon.

1. BUSINESS CARDS

    The use of quality cards to obtain new patients has been discussed earlier. This equally applies to keeping the ones you have. It is good to leave your card with every new patient. Although some will lose it others will treat it like a club membership card – the 'if ever you are in trouble you can phone this number' club.

2. RECEIPTS

    It is strongly recommended that you make a habit of giving all patients receipts. You will need a receipt book for places like nursing homes where the staff are handling patients' affairs, so make a practice of using them for everyone. There are several very cheap series to choose from with two receipts to a page which are ideal. You can stamp them with your name, address and telephone number, or for ease use Able-labels or a similar product. They help you to keep patients because:

    a) Firstly – it *looks* professional. The chiropodist who simply asks for cash which he stuffs into a pocket, could be a 'moonlighter'. But *you* give receipts. *You* are in legitimate practice. (It underlines why yours is a proper professional fee.) *You* are the person to trust!

    b) Secondly – while many people mislay business and appointment cards, for some reason they often hoard receipts like they were bank notes! So your telephone number is always on hand. If you use the back of the receipt to give date and time of next appointment then this saves on appointment cards as well.

3. PATIENT LETTERS

    Paper is cheap. Your time is not. There are many opportunities to leave instruction letters with patients for their reference after you have long gone. This can be of great value to them, since verbal instructions often go in one ear and straight out the other. It can be of great value to you, since there, overprinted or stuck on the bottom, tastefully but unmistakably, are your practice details.

Patient letters could include:

a)   the diabetic foot;
b)   treatment of athlete's foot;
c)   verrucae treatment and aftercare;
d)   footwear and feet;
e)   care of your appliance/silicone/insole;
f)   proper nail cutting;
g)   etc.

You may get leaflets through your professional association, or you may produce them yourself. If you burst into prose, remember not to be too erudite. Instructions have to be simple and clear. The limited vocabulary of tabloid journalism is effective with most people. The finished product then has to be a comfortable print size for elderly patients to read.

4.   REMINDER LETTERS

When I get a six month reminder letter from my dentist – I go! If he forgets to send me one, I wait until something drops out and it hurts!

A simple letter after six months works wonders at reminding the more casual patient that you are their chiropodist. For example, under your letter heading you might say:

SIX MONTHS CHECK-UP NOTICE

As the regular care of your feet is important, and it is now six months since your last treatment, may I respectfully suggest that a further appointment would be beneficial at this time.

Please write or telephone for a home visit.

Sincerely

(signed)

To organise reminder letters is a very simple operation. Ultimately it is also very cheap. Just one patient telephoning will have paid for a considerable number of stamps.

Once a month, or whenever, all you need to do is quickly flick through the cards in your patient file to check who has not telephoned. For those due a letter, you mark on a top corner of the card the month and year their reminder is sent. Then when the patient comes back to you, you simply cross through the month and year reference. The advantage of having such a note on the top of the card is that when your file is bursting with patient details, those who are currently 'dead' are immediately obvious, and you do not have to waste time looking at these cards. But it is surprising how many will appreciate the memory jog it gave them and will come back to you as a direct result.

If for space reasons you need to have a clear-out of cards of patients not seen for several years, then the record on the top of the card makes it a very easy exercise to do. (Of course by clear-out we do *not* mean the dustbin, but removal to another place of storage for at least seven years.)

Those who spend many hours saving time with computers will no doubt be dismissive of the primitive nature of the above operation, and will have something highly technical worked out to do the job. If so, then fine. But just remember that if you do not have the permission of *every* patient to be on your database you are in fact breaking the law.

5. OTHER CIRCULARS

Even if there is no response to a reminder letter (you were such a good chiropodist – you cured them ...) there can still be opportunities to send a circular to selected patients after a reasonable interval.

Some private health insurance companies now provide leaflets advertising help with chiropody fees, and are only too happy for you to distribute them. Overstamped with your details they are another tactful reminder that you exist, and that the former patient might have need of you. Again, as soon as just one patient has made an appointment this will have paid for quite a mail-out. From then on, it is all to your advantage.

At the end of the day remember that all the advertising technique in the world will not succeed, if all it does is to remind a person of an experience they would rather forget! So as stressed at the outset, do your best for each patient, give them the time, the attention, and the full benefit of your expertise. Then you will keep them.

Accounts

"In this world nothing can be said to be certain – except death and taxes," said Benjamin Franklin. Leaving the Grim Reaper aside for the moment, taxation is one essential subject the newly qualified, self-employed chiropodist must get to grips with!

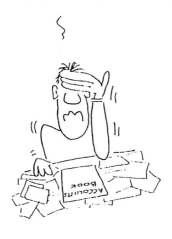

Sadly, many small businesses bite the dust because people who may be very good at their trade or profession just cannot handle the paperwork. Make sure this is not you! With just a little care a fledgling chiropodist should be able to handle their own accounts without the need to employ an accountant.

For specific questions about what is required you will find a visit to the local tax office very practical. They can supply up-to-date information and current literature for the self-employed on what is now called 'self assessment'. This covers both income tax and national insurance contributions which are handled by the same office. If there is anything about your particular situation that you do not understand, then ask. They are normally very helpful. In other words, what follows may be vague in certain details and is hedged about with the usual disclaimers.. But it is an attempt to describe a simple way of accounting for *absolute beginners*.

Tax for the self-employed

If you work for an employer under the Pay-As-You-Earn scheme (PAYE) that is what you do! After personal allowances are calculated the required income tax and national insurance contribution is deducted from each wage packet. It is money you never actually see.

When you are a self-employed tax-payer you do see the money, because you pay *after* you earn. This means that you had better be careful not to *spend* as you earn – not all of it anyway! Your income may well fluctuate over the year but it is the annual amount that matters. Your tax bill and national insurance will be based on your total profits. (How these are calculated will follow.) You need to have things worked out in sufficient detail so that, first, your accounts are accurate and reflect only what you are liable to pay in tax, and second, that you haven't already spent it all on those three weeks in Tenerife before the bill comes.

Your accounting year

You can start your own accounting year from whenever you like. In theory, if you start up in practice on November 1st, for example, that would be the start of your accounting year. So your accounts would be drawn up for the year ending October 31st.

However, it is quite in order to change the start of your accounting year. The tax office does not like your doing this too often, and no matter how you juggle it you will still get the bill eventually! But they will allow you to adjust you starting date if you choose, and thereby have a longer or shorter 'year' on the one occasion. In this event your tax liability is simply worked out on a percentage basis for the length of the one odd period.

So with this freedom of choice, when should you start your accounting year? When established, it can make sense to have your accounting year the same as the calendar year, starting on January 1st and ending on December 31st. Major records like appointments diaries will normally run for this period. The self assessment form will be sent out to you after the end of the tax year on April 5th, and you will then have several months before you need return it. So ending your accounting year on December 31st should give you sufficient time to get it all together.

The only danger with such extended deadlines is that you might slide into the 'out of sight, out of mind' syndrome – you first procrastinate on the paperwork, and then mislay the forms. Not a good idea! We will return to these forms later.

Three line accounts

For small businesses with a low turnover the tax office will accept what are called three line accounts. (Check the forms for the current ceiling on gross income.) However, even if applicable for you at present you would still be well advised to keep more detailed accounts for yourself. Someone's law suggests that if you don't, you could be the one person in a thousand some perverse official decides to investigate.

Three line accounts mean what they say – three lines. They are as follows:

Line one: Your total gross income or turnover.

Line two: Your total allowable expenses.

Line three: Taking line two away from line one will give you your profits (or losses) – what, at the end of the day, you can actually say you have earned as income.

You will then be taxed on your profits, after personal allowances have been considered. So, as already stressed, be sure to put sufficient aside to pay this bill. We hope you are well on your way to becoming a chiropody tycoon, but you do not want a tax bill when going through a temporary slump unless you have squirreled away sufficient funds (earning good interest one hopes) to meet it. When you have done your accounts and know your 'profits' it is reasonably easy to work out what your bill should be.

Of course you may have few patients to begin with, and extra expenses stocking up with supplies, and you may escape a tax bill the first time around – but you still need to have the pieces of paper and a little bit of bookwork to prove this.

If your turnover is over the limit for three line accounts, basically the tax office will want a lot more detail about your expenses.

In a sense there is a fourth line with these simple accounts, for what are called capital allowances. These are large expenses which can be set against more than one year. We will deal with these later.

Let us now run through the basic three lines in more detail, and how we can ensure we get it right.

First, our total gross income or turnover. How do you keep track of this?

One way is to use your appointments book to record what sums you take from patients. In addition, or instead, you can use the carbon entries in a receipt book. We have already extolled the virtues of giving receipts as a means of advertising and keeping patients. But for accounting purposes, with a receipt book it is very easy at the end of the day, week, or month to establish what you have taken. You can then enter the results in an accounts book at intervals as it suits you. If you leave it all until the end of the year and panic – it can still be done!

If you number the counterfoils in your receipt books you can check very easily how many patients you are treating weekly or monthly, and this can be helpful in identifying the exact progress of the practice, along with such anomalies as seasonal variations in casual patients in some areas – e.g. they all want their feet done before Christmas and before holidays and they all are broke afterwards!

After you have entered the details in your accounts book, still keep the receipts. In fact keep all the bits of paper. Chiro's law states that if you don't, you will be the one person in a thousand that the Inland Revenue decides to do a spot check on!

Our second line is the total *allowable* expenses incurred in the practice. You really *must* keep all the bits of paper here. You need to be able to prove that any expense has in fact occurred. Some expenses can be claimed in their entirety, e.g. chiropody materials, postages for the practice, advertising, professional subscriptions and insurances. For other expenses you can claim a proportion, e.g. a telephone or motor vehicle that has part business and part private use. On the basis that you use your home to store supplies, take calls, work out your accounts, etc. a small percentage of your household expenses can be claimed. For the exact percentages in your case it would be well to get general agreement with your local tax office.

How do you keep track of all these details? The easiest way is to use an analysis book or a pad of analysis paper, obtainable from any good stationer.

As illustrated above this has a number of columns which you can use to record each type of expense. It is good to keep the different expenses separate in this way since some will only be percentages at the end of the year. It is also useful to be able to be able to check annual expenditure on specific things like advertising, supplies, stationery, etc.

It is better to have too many columns in your book than too few. In your first year different types of expenses may occur, and if you have too few columns you are going to run out of space. To play safe have at least 12 columns, even if they do not all get used.

Let us now examine part of a sample completed page.

DATE	DETAILS	RECEIPT No.	GROSS	MOTORING	POSTAGE STATIONERY	FEE
JAN 2	PETROL	1	22 00	22 00		
3	POSTAGE	2	4 50		4 50	
5	CAR SERVICE	3	64 50	64 50		
7	CHIRO JOURNAL SUB	4	32 00			32
7	PETROL	5	22 00	22 00		
9	CHIRO SUPPLIES	6	42 80			
12	TELEPHONE	7	90 40			

Working across the page, you first put the date and then use the wide column to write in the purchase details, petrol, stamps, chiropody supplies, etc.

You must obtain receipts for every purchase. It is very practical to number them for easy reference throughout the year and put the

64

receipt number down in the next small column. If you want to refer to a specific receipt at any time you can then find it straight away. Even if you thrive on muddle, make a practice of *always* putting receipts in one place. It can be special envelopes month by month, a special drawer, a shoebox, or whatever — but whatever you do, *do not lose them!*

If you are using a business account for purchases it can also be very useful to include the cheque number in your accounts along with the receipt number. This is a double check that the money has been spent as stated.

Now we come to the actual analysis columns which are numbered. In column one under the heading 'Gross' or 'Total' put down the total amount you have spent. Then in each succeeding column you list the *type* of expense, and also put the amount spent down *again* under the relevant heading.

The headings could include:

Motor vehicle
Postage and stationery
Professional fees, subscriptions and insurances
Clothing
Subsistence and travel
Telephone
Advertising
Household
Business account bank charges
Chiropody expenses

At the end of any set period of time you can add up each individual column. Column one will tell you the straight total of all expenditure. Then the other columns will 'analyse' where exactly it all went. So much on stationery, so much on insurance, etc.

If you then add up all the individual totals at the bottom of the page they should come to the grand total obtained by adding up column one. If you are still with me, this is quite a good check that you have not punched the wrong button on the calculator somewhere along the line.

Most of the headings are self-explanatory. Unless you have an account with one garage by far the greatest number of entries will be the running costs of your vehicle. You will need a receipt every time you buy petrol etc. If the car is used other than for chiropody you may need to keep a mileage log to establish fairly the amount of business use and personal use. On your final accounts you adjust accordingly.

Your professional dues will include your association membership, your practice insurance, and also any other directly related subscriptions. Most of the chiropody/podiatry journals are available on subscription to non-members of associations, and when starting out it is good to be as well read as possible.

If you attend a seminar, or have additional training, which involves rail travel and the need for some accommodation, these expenses should be entered under 'Subsistence and Travel'.

If you have a business account then your bank charges are a deductable expense. Your business account will always cost you more to run than an ordinary account, so it is wise to keep it just for business use, and with your hand on your heart you can then claim all the bank charges. As an extra check if receipts go missing, you may want to have your cheques returned to you with your bank statements. On seeing how much your bank will charge for this service, you may not!

Finally, at the end of the year you work out the percentage for those expenses you cannot claim in full. It might look like this:

Item	Gross	%	Net
Motoring	2683.35	83%	2227.18
Postage/stationery	90.64		90.64
Professional fees/insur.	142.00		142.00
Telephone	467.65	80%	374.12
Advertising	258.50		258.50
Allow. household	1122.52	10%	112.25
Business a/c charges	103.50		103.50
Chiropody supplies	452.60		452.60
Total allowable expenses:			3760.79

You can now complete line two of your three line accounts – total allowable expenses.

If you take line two (allowable expenses) away from line one (gross taking) you get line three – what you are actually worth!

Capital allowances

There just remains the matter of capital allowances. Certain items purchased just cannot be put down as expenses for the one year. A new vehicle or a large item of equipment will be used for several years, and so are allowed over a longer period. You will be permitted to claim a certain amount for depreciation each year. It is wise to check with the tax office , but for many items it is 25% per annum. So if, for example, you purchase a very small domiciliary case for £100, in the first year you can claim 25% of this as a capital allowance, namely £25. The next year you can claim a further 25% but note that this would not be another £25 but rather 25% of the balance of £75 – which would work out at £18.75. The third year the residue would be £56.25 (£75 less £18.75) and your 25% would now be £14.06. Eventually you change the case for a new one, or write off the last remaining balance.

Comparisons

The taxman is only interested in what you have earned over the year, but if you want to divide your line three 'profits' by fifty-two, you can see how much you earn each week on average as a domiciliary chiropodist.

Of course, you hopefully don't plan to work for 52 weeks a year. To make a valid comparison with having an employer (perhaps in a previous life) do not forget your holidays.

When an employed person takes annual leave, he still gets his basic wage. His employer pays. He gets three or four weeks wages or more for doing absolutely nothing! But when you take time off – you pay! With your own business it comes out of *your* time and *your* earnings. So you need to earn considerably *more* each working week than someone with an employer if you are to be as financially well off, and be able to take time off too.

It is an equation that many starting down the self-employed road do not immediately realise.

Finally, what should you do when a little after April 5th you get your first taste of the Inland Revenue's self assessment form?

The straight answer is, fill out something on it and return it! Do not leave it. A forgotten tax return will not just fade away, it will come back and haunt you.

People in Britain just love filling out forms. Yeah – and pigs might fly. In spite of plain English campaigns, the designers of forms seem intent on exposing your inability to unravel the inner workings of the official mind.

So probably the very first thing you should do when it all lands on the doormat, is get the forms photocopied. If you start off using the originals, you will invariably make a mistake near the beginning, which will be carried through all the subsequent calculations and mess the whole thing up. Scribble over photocopies with impunity, but leave the originals until you are really sure what you are doing.

In completing a self assessment tax return there are three basic deadlines to consider. (The tax office will give you the actual dates for these currently in operation.)

The first deadline is for the tax office to do all the work. If you can make this deadline all you need to really do is supply your three line accounts, along with any other income that needs to be declared – then the Inland Revenue will calculate your tax bill. There is no guarantee they will get their sums right, but they will outline *how* they reached the figure being demanded – which is a good starting point to check. Once you have checked their calculations through one year you may feel enthusiastic about doing it yourself in the future. Or maybe not.

If, by choice or default, you miss deadline one the second deadline is for *you* to do all the work. You complete your basic accounts and then follow directions on the forms, going from box to box like a demented board game. Personal allowances and a sliding scale of National Insurance contributions are amongst the delights awaiting you. There is obviously no guarantee *you* will get the sums right, but the Revenue will correct your figures as needed and tell you where you went wrong.

Obviously you will need to keep a photocopy of your completed form as sent to understand all this several weeks or months down the line.

If you miss deadlines one and two you are in trouble. "Form, what form?" and "It's in the post" cut little ice. You become subject to an automatic pain in the wallet. There is a fixed fine penalty and yet another date – deadline three. By deadline three you must still produce the completed forms *and* pay the fine – or there is another fine on top! And all this before you've even had the bill for the income tax you owe. Believe me – they don't give up. It just gets worse.

So don't become one of those statistics who habitually postpone the job, miss the first deadline, get flummoxed trying to work out the complexities of the form and miss the second deadline, and get a fine on top of everything else.

In conclusion then, you really do need to get to grips with your basic accounts and accounting responsibilities as a self-employed chiropodist. Number things. Don't lose them. Keep the paperwork up-to-date. Get the papers in on time. You will have that smug satisfaction of watching all those TV advertisements for poor souls who are still desperately rummaging around for two year old receipts, knowing that YOU have done it right. You may still have a nasty shock when the bill arrives, but you can check it through and if necessary raise some dust before actually parting with any money. This will be required in two instalments over the next year, unless the amount is very small and one payment only is required.

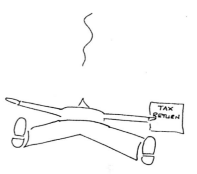

Eventually of course you are going to earn a sufficient amount to employ a team of accountants and tax advisors, before retiring to the South of France and forgetting all about the wonderful world of chiropody. That, however, must be the subject of another book.